POCKET GUIDES

CW00924634

RADIOTHERAPY IN CLINICAL PRACTICE

A unique series of pocket-sized books designed to help healthcare students

"All the information was clear and concise, this book is exactly what I was looking for." ★★★★★

"A great little guide. All the basic information needed to have a quick reference." ★★★★★

"A very useful, well-written and practical pocket book." ★★★★★

"Written by students for students. A must for any student about to head on placement." ★★★★★

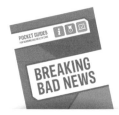

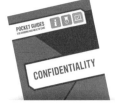

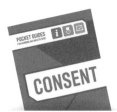

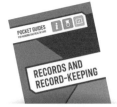

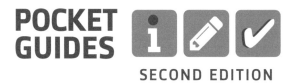

POCKET GUIDES

SECOND EDITION

RADIOTHERAPY IN CLINICAL PRACTICE

Lucy Austin
2013 Society of Radiographers Student of the Year

Teresa Howe
University Hospitals Bristol and Weston NHS Foundation Trust

Sian Jamison
University Hospitals Bristol and Weston NHS Foundation Trust

Lantern

ISBN 9781914962226

First published in 2024 by Lantern Publishing Ltd
First edition published in 2014 (as *Pocket Guide for
Radiotherapy in Clinical Practice: A handbook for
first-year students during clinical placement*)

Lantern Publishing Limited, The Old Hayloft, Vantage
Business Park, Bloxham Road, Banbury OX16 9UX, UK
www.lanternpublishing.com

British Library Cataloguing in Publication Data
A catalogue record for this book is available from the British Library

The authors and publisher have made every attempt to ensure
the content of this book is up to date and accurate. However,
healthcare knowledge and information is changing all the time
so the reader is advised to double-check any information in
this text on drug usage, treatment procedures, the use of
equipment, etc. to confirm that it complies with the latest safety
recommendations, standards of practice and legislation, as well as
local Trust policies and procedures. Students are advised to check
with their tutor and/or practice supervisor before carrying out
any of the procedures in this textbook.

Typeset by Medlar Publishing Solutions Pvt Ltd, India
Printed and bound in the UK

Last digit is the print number: 10 9 8 7 6 5 4 3 2 1

Personal information

Name: . . . .

Mobile number: . . . .

Address during placement:. . . . .

. . . .

. . . .

. . . .

PLACEMENT DETAILS

Hospital: . . . .

Hospital address:. . . . .

. . . .

. . . .

. . . .

Phone number: . . . .

Link lecturer: . . . .

CONTACT IN CASE OF EMERGENCY

Name: . . . .

Mobile number: . . . .

Home/work number:. . . . .

Contents

Preface to the second edition. vii

Abbreviations ix

1. The correct uniform 1
2. Radiotherapy treatment room. 2
3. Immobilisation devices 3
4. Hospital bins. 6
5. Top tips for your radiotherapy placement 7
6. Sharps bin. 8
7. How to make a permanent skin mark (tattoo)
   when in pre-treatment. 9
8. Effective communication 10
9. First day chat 11
10. Couch moves. 12
11. Isocentre calculations 13
12. Laser positioning 14
13. Before setting up the patient 16
14. How to align the tattoos 17
15. Naming different beam angles 18
16. How can cancer spread? 19
17. Typical radiotherapy techniques. 21
    17.1 Radical prostate. 21
    17.2 Radical breast 23
    17.3 Radical bladder 25
    17.4 Radical lung 27
    17.5 Radical rectum. 29
18. Tolerance doses 31
19. What is SABR?. 32

20. What is brachytherapy? 33
21. What is electron treatment? 34
22. What is orthovoltage and superficial
X-ray therapy? 35
23. What is IGRT? 37
24. What is IMRT? 40
25. Radiotherapy treatment pathway 41
26. What is hormone therapy? 42
27. What is immunotherapy? 43
28. What is chemotherapy? 44
29. Chemotherapy side-effects 45
30. Radiotherapy side-effects 46
31. Blood values 50
32. Radiotherapy manufacturers 51
33. Basic anatomy 52
34. Vertebral levels 54
35. Manual handling 56
36. Infection control 57
37. Basic life support 58
38. The recovery position 59
39. Medical terminology 60

Preface to the second editio

This pocket guide was originally produced by Lucy Austin as part of her dissertation. This book incorporates some basic concepts along with more complex areas which students often find difficult to master initially. Lucy received external recognition in the form of the "Student of the year" award from our professional body, The College of Radiographers, in 2013.

Since the original publication of this guide, there have been many advances in radiotherapy. We have updated this guide to reflect changes in practice. As radiotherapy is always changing, we have tried to keep the information general – it is important to check department protocols at each placement site.

We hope this book helps to introduce you to your first placement, and wish you all the best in the departments!

Teresa Howe
Sian Jamisor

Abbreviations

ABC	active breathing control
AP	anteroposterior
ART	adaptive radiotherapy
BCC	basal cell carcinoma
BED	biological effective dose
BEV	beam's eye view
Bx	biopsy
Ca	cancer or carcinoma
CBC	complete blood count (same as FBC)
CBCT	cone beam CT
CFRT	conformal radiotherapy
CHART	continuous, hyperfractionated accelerated radiotherapy
CNS	central nervous system or Clinical Nurse Specialist
CRT	chemoradiotherapy
CSF	cerebrospinal fluid
CT	computed tomography
CTV	clinical target volume
DIBH	deep inspiration breath hold (see also VBH)
DOB	date of birth
DRR	digital reconstructed radiograph
EBRT	external beam radiotherapy
EPID	electronic portal imaging device
FBC	full blood count (same as CBC)
FSD	Focus-Skin-Distance
GTV	gross tumour volume
H&H	haemoglobin and haematocrit
HAD	hospital anxiety depression scale

> Confusion in the use of abbreviations has been cited as the reason for some clinical incidents. Therefore you should use these abbreviations with caution and only in line with local Trusts' Clinical Governance recommendations which vary between departments!

HPV	human papilloma virus
ICC	intercostal catheter
IGRT	image-guided radiotherapy
IMRT	intensity-modulated radiotherapy
IORT	intraoperative radiotherapy
IVC	intravenous catheter
LFT	liver function test
MLC	multi-leaf collimator
MRI	magnetic resonance imaging
MSA	mental state assessment
MSU	mid-stream urine
MTD	maximum tolerated dose
NHL	non-Hodgkin's lymphoma
NSCLC	non small cell lung cancer
OAR	organ at risk
PA	posteroanterior
PCI	prophylactic cranial irradiation
PET	positron emission tomography
PS	performance status
PSA	prostate-specific antigen
PTV	planning target volume
RapidArc	VMAT on Varian linacs
RR	relative risk
SABR	stereotactic ablative body radiotherapy
SCC	squamous cell carcinoma
SCLC	small cell lung cancer
SGRT	surface guided radiotherapy
SPECT	single photon emission computed tomography
SRT	stereotactic radiotherapy

SSD	source skin distance
TBI	total body irradiation
TCT	transitional cell tumours
TLD	thermo-luminescent dosemeter
TNM	tumour, nodes, metastases
UA	urinalysis
VBH	voluntary breath hold (*see also* DIBH)
VMAT	volumetric arc therapy
WBC	white blood cell
XVI	X-ray volumetric imaging (CBCT on Elekta)

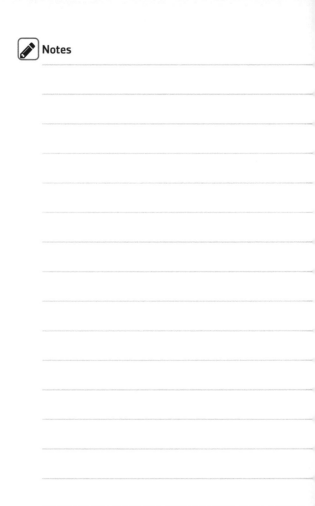

Notes

The correct uniform

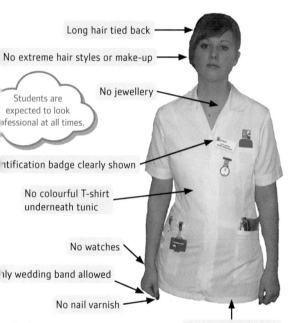

Long hair tied back

No extreme hair styles or make-up

No jewellery

Students are expected to look professional at all times.

Identification badge clearly shown

No colourful T-shirt underneath tunic

No watches

Only wedding band allowed

No nail varnish

Clean, ironed uniform

Shoes should be plain black with toes covered

You are NOT allowed to work without a **TLD**!

Equipment needed:

- Pens – red, blue, black
- Permanent marker pen
- Pencil
- 15 cm metal ruler
- Fob watch (optional)
- Notebook (included at the end of this pocket guide)
- Small calculator
- Film card (provided)

1

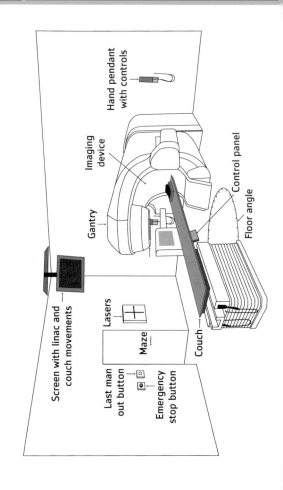

Hand pendant with controls

Imaging device

Gantry

Control panel

Floor angle

Screen with linac and couch movements

Lasers

Maze

Couch

Last man out button

Emergency stop button

Immobilisation devices

These are some of the immobilisation devices used to stabilise the patient. This is so that they maintain their position throughout treatment. These devices will vary between departments.

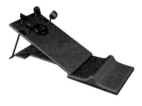

Breast board
This is used to treat the breast. The patient's head lies on a support (not always doughnut-shaped) and the arms are raised into the cup-shaped holders.

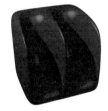

Ankle/foot support
This is used to stabilise the patient's feet, and is typically used for pelvis patients.

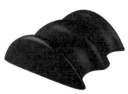

Knee support
This is used to help the patient maintain their position by supporting their knees and back; this pad is used on most treatments.

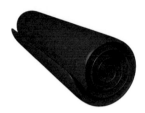

Thin foam
Typically used for patients who may struggle to lie on the hard carbon fibre treatment bed.

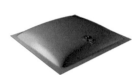

Vac bag
This reusable bag contains lots of small polystyrene balls which are moulded around the patient. A vacuum pump then sucks all of the air out, making it firm, and an imprint is then made of the patient. This can then be used for each fraction.

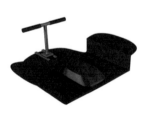

Wing board
This is used to treat the chest. The patient holds the T-bar or a U-shaped bar whilst their head lies on the head pad. Sometimes a Vac bag is placed inside this for additional support. The patient's elbows rest on the wings or in arm support.

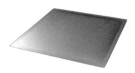

Bolus
It is placed over the patient's skin and secured using tape. Bolus is used to bring the isodose up to the skin surface. The material is tissue equivalent to the skin density.

Wax
This can be used to create a uniform block. It is placed or shaped around the treatment area, for example the nose for electron treatments. This makes the dose distribution more homogeneous.

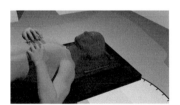

Head mask
Head masks are individually shaped for each patient. The sides of the mask are moulded around the face and secured using either clips or blocks. Claustrophobic patients can struggle greatly with this device, and sometimes a bite block is required to immobilise the tongue. The mask can extend to below the shoulders. This device is used on patients with head/neck or upper lung cancers.

Hospitals have colour-coded bins to determine what type of waste should be put in them.

It is important that you dispose of any waste in the appropriate bin.

Colour of bin	Use	Example
Black	Domestic waste	Packaging
Yellow	Hazardous and infectious waste	Gloves, aprons, items with blood on
Yellow with black line	Offensive waste	Incontinence pads
Purple	Cytotoxic waste	Chemotherapy drugs
Orange	Infectious waste	Dressings

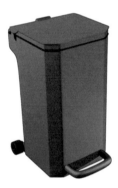

Any paper containing patient information needs to be shredded separately. There is a separate bin/bag for this.

Top tips for your radiotherapy placement

1. First impressions last, so it's important to be professional and punctual at all times.
2. If you are required to undertake any research or paperwork during your placement, ensure you begin it as soon as possible to allow for checking and alterations by a practice educator.
3. Always ask if you don't understand or if you are unsure about what is happening – you are there to learn.
4. Think about any desirable experiences as soon as possible, so you can get them organised more quickly, and make the most of your time available in the department.
5. You may be expected to do mental arithmetic on the treatment floor. If you struggle with this you may want to practise beforehand or use a pocket calculator.
6. Be comfortable saying to a patient *"Sorry, I am a student, let me just ask/get my colleague"*.
7. Try to have a walk around the department and familiarise yourself. The quicker you know your way around, the easier it is to settle.

Notes

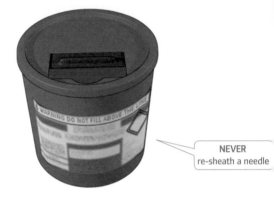

NEVER
re-sheath a needle

ANY sharp instruments must be placed in a yellow/orange 'sharps bin' after use, for incineration.

Remember to partially close the lid after each use but do not fully close the lid as it will permanently lock. Only fully close the bin when it is filled to the max line, to avoid a costly wastage of materials.

When using sharp materials such as a needle you should have a sharps bin within reach in order to dispose of the instrument immediately.

Do not leave any sharp materials for someone else to clear.

Do not walk around with a needle or sharp instrument. If you need to put the needle down, simply dispose of it and use a new one.

Do not use any sterilised equipment which is already opened – you do not know if it has already been used!

How to make a permanent skin mark (tattoo) when in pre-treatment

Not all students will be able to tattoo the patient in their first year, but if you do here are some helpful tips. Remember, only undertake this procedure if you feel confident and fully understand the process.

- Stay calm at all times; this will help the patient stay relaxed.
- Take your time and do not rush.
- Ensure you are supervised, as a qualified member of staff needs to sign that the tattoo has been completed successfully.
- Ensure you have everything you need BEFORE you start.
- Check the patient has consented to having the tattoo and explain the procedure.
- Bring tray/trolley with equipment to the patient.
- Wipe the skin clean with an antibacterial wipe.
- DO NOT use an already opened/unsheathed needle.
- Wear gloves/apron AND wash hands before and after.
- Pierce the skin at an 45° angle, then lift slightly to allow the ink to flow under the skin.
- Either syringe ink into the needle beforehand or dab ink onto the pierced skin using a new cotton bud.
- Place needle immediately into sharps bin once finished. If needle needs to be put down, bin it, and use a new one.
- Wipe excess ink from skin, check the tattoo has been clearly made and dispose of equipment using appropriate bins.

> As departments move to surface-guided radiotherapy, tattoos may not be required. Ensure you read local guidance before undertaking any permanent skin mark-up.

Take time to listen to your patient!

Do not use medical language which will confuse the patient.

Patients may be very anxious; talk in a calm manner at all times.

Be aware of who can overhear your conversation with the patient.

Appear welcoming and approachable.

Maintain eye contact which is comfortable for you and your patient.

Body language is important when engaging your patient – hand gestures can help illustrate a point.

It is important to look interested in what the patient is saying to you.

Reference: Easton, S. (2008) *An Introduction to Radiography*. Churchill Livingstone, pp. 23–40.

First day chat

Six key points to remember when treating the patient for the first time:

1. Check the patient has signed the consent form and still consents to treatment. A pregnancy form must be completed by all females aged 10–55 years. This must be done BEFORE the patient starts their treatment.
2. Identify the patient using 3 forms of positive identification. Learn your placement department's procedure. It could be full name, date of birth, address, area being treated.
3. Make sure the patient understands any side-effects they may experience and explain that these will not happen immediately. It is usually at least a week before they may start to notice any changes.
4. Ask the patient if they have any questions or concerns before they start treatment. Explain any terminology the patient may not be familiar with on their appointment list, such as machine name and what the review appointments are. It would be good to mention that the patient will not see or feel anything during the treatment.
5. Run through what the patient will expect during their treatment. For example, the noises the machine makes.
6. Explain that the radiographers can still see and hear the patient at all times so we can stop the machine immediately if there is a problem.

> A relaxed patient can be set up more quickly and smoothly

10 | Couch moves

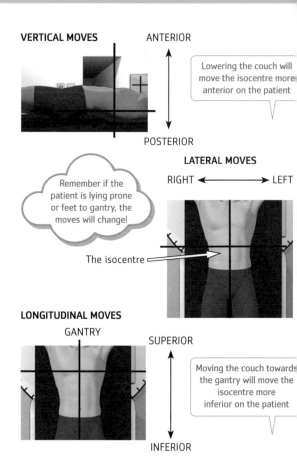

VERTICAL MOVES

ANTERIOR

Lowering the couch will move the isocentre more anterior on the patient

POSTERIOR

LATERAL MOVES

RIGHT ← → LEFT

Remember if the patient is lying prone or feet to gantry, the moves will change!

The isocentre

LONGITUDINAL MOVES

GANTRY

SUPERIOR

Moving the couch towards the gantry will move the isocentre more inferior on the patient

INFERIOR

Isocentre calculations

Once a patient has been lined up to the tattoos, there may be some alterations to the couch. This is to move the planning target volume to the isocentre.

This only applies for supine – head first

Move to be made	Couch orientation
Superior 'Sup'	**Subtract:** from the <u>longitudinal</u> value
Inferior 'Inf'	**Add:** on to the <u>longitudinal</u> value
Posterior 'Post'	**Subtract:** from the <u>vertical</u> value
Anterior 'Ant'	**Add:** on to <u>vertical</u> value
Left	**Subtract:** from the <u>lateral</u> value
Right	**Add:** on to the <u>lateral</u> value

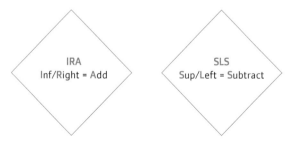

IRA
Inf/Right = Add

SLS
Sup/Left = Subtract

The position of the lasers in relation to the tattoo is often stated throughout the set-up process. We are aiming to get the tattoo in the centre of the cross (isocentre) on both sides of the patient.

Below is a step-by-step process of understanding what is being stated.

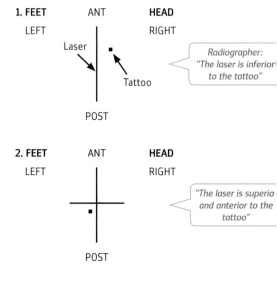

1. FEET   ANT   **HEAD**

LEFT   RIGHT

Laser

Tattoo

POST

Radiographer: "The laser is inferior to the tattoo"

2. FEET   ANT   **HEAD**

LEFT   RIGHT

POST

"The laser is superio and anterior to the tattoo"

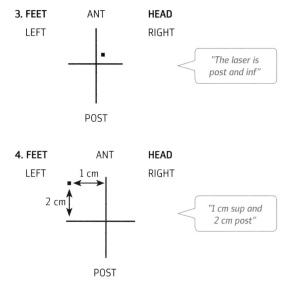

This explains where the laser is in relation to the tattoo. In some departments this could be the other way around; for example, the position of the tattoo could be described in relation to where the laser is. You should clarify this when you first start working on the treatment unit, to avoid confusion.

Notes

Before we start aligning the tattoos with the lasers, there are a few things to remember.

- Has the first day chat been undertaken, if it is the patient's first treatment? (see *Chapter 9*).
- Have you correctly identified your patient?
- Have you asked how the patient is today? They may be worried about something or have some questions. It is important to check with your patient that they are not struggling with any side-effects that we can help with.
- Have you reminded the patient that they need to wait after treatment to see the doctor/review radiographer or have any bloodwork? (if applicable).
- Has the patient removed the item(s) of clothing required for the treatment area before getting onto the couch?
- Once the patient is lying on the bed you should check that they are lying straight. This is done by making sure the sagittal laser (laser going down the length of the couch) is running through the middle of the sternum. Standing at the end of the couch will also help you to see if the patient is straight.

Once you have done this, the next step will be aligning the tattoos with the lasers.

With SGRT, there may be no tattoos, but having the patient lying straight is essential for reproducibility.

 Notes

_____

_____

_____

How to align the tattoos

Before any shifts can be done, the two lateral tattoos (the tattoos on the patient's sides) need to be level. In order to do this, we move the bed so the isocentre is on one of the lateral tattoos (the isocentre is where the lasers make a cross). Now one tattoo is aligned, we need to move the patient so both lateral tattoos are in the centre of the cross (isocentre). Here are some tips on how we can manipulate the patient in order to get the tattoos level with each other.

- Only rotate the patient about half the way you want, otherwise you will rotate too much in one direction.
- Don't be afraid to ask the patient to help. For example, if a pelvic tattoo is superior, you can move the patient's leg for minor changes, or ask the patient to stretch down their leg for large movements.
- For 'sup' and 'inf' movements involving chest/breast patients, try moving the patient's upper arm and raising the elbow slightly. This will adjust the tattoo more superior. The opposite will move the tattoo more inferior.
- For 'ant' and 'post' movements place your hands on either side of the patient and rotate one side down. Rotating the patient this way will make the tattoo on the opposite side more anterior so the radiographer will raise the bed.
- Remember it takes time and lots of practice. Don't worry if you move the patient in the wrong direction; this can be easily corrected by trying a different movement.
- Always be proactive to make sure you get lots of practice.

15 | Naming different beam angles

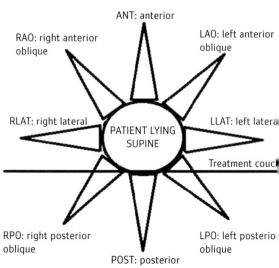

ANT: anterior

LAO: left anterior oblique

RAO: right anterior oblique

RLAT: right lateral

PATIENT LYING SUPINE

LLAT: left lateral

Treatment couch

RPO: right posterior oblique

LPO: left posterior oblique

POST: posterior

 Note

> With VMAT treatment, the beams will be made up of arcs, typically clockwise or counterclockwise.

 Notes

How can cancer spread?

When a cancer spreads away from the primary cancer it is known to be 'metastatic' and the secondary cancer that forms is called a 'metastasis' or 'metastases' for more than one. There are five main routes of spread:

Bloodstream

Usually sarcomas. A cancer cell can get stuck in the thin-walled capillary and grow.

Lymphatic system

Carcinomas usually spread through the lymphatic system to local lymph nodes first. For example, breast cancer can spread to axillary lymph nodes.

Direct invasion

Where the cancer invades neighbouring tissues.

Implantation

Where the cancer is spread through medical instruments or naturally. For example, during surgery some cells may be left in the scar tissue or along the ureters to the bladder.

Transcoelomic

Spread across body cavities, this can happen during surgery or direct invasion.

✏️ **Notes**

_____

_____

_____

_____

_____

_____

_____

_____

_____

_____

_____

Typical radiotherapy techniques

17.1 Radical prostate

(Techniques will vary between departments.)

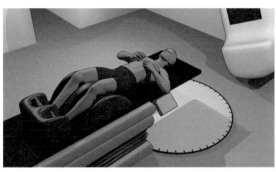

Typical beam arrangement

IMRT or VMAT moving 360° around the patient.

Non-IMRT patients may have a four-field box arrangement.

Patient position

Supine, head to gantry, hands on chest.

Treatment preparation

Organ motion can be controlled by bladder and rectum preparation prior to each treatment.

Empty rectum (e.g. the patient may be asked to use a micro enema prior to each treatment) and to have a comfortable full bladder. This may be department-dependent. Please check the department's protocol.

Immobilisation devices

Stocks or Vac bag to secure the patient's feet, along with a knee support.

Typical prescriptions

60 Gy in 20# over 4 weeks (prostate only).

74 Gy in 37# over 7.5 weeks (prostate plus pelvic lymph nodes).

66 Gy in 33# over 6.5 weeks (prostate bed).

Notes

17.2 Radical breast

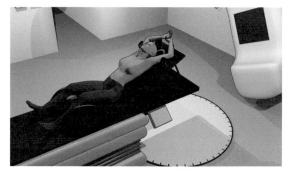

Typical beam arrangement

Two beams in a tangential field pair arrangement. If there is lymph node involvement, an anterior supraclavicular field may be added.

Patient position

Patient is supine and sitting up slightly on the angled breast board with one or both arms up. Knees are slightly bent. Some departments provide special breast gowns to maintain patient dignity.

Immobilisation devices

A breast board with attachable head support and arm rests. A knee support helps prevent the patient from sliding down the board.

> Breast boards can get very cold. Putting a pillowcase on the board can help with this.

Typical prescriptions

40 Gy in 15# over 3 weeks (breast plus lymph nodes).

26 Gy in 5# over 1 week (breast only).

Breast/breast plus lymph nodes on the left-hand side may be treated using a technique called deep inspiration breath hold (DIBH). Holding a deep breath allows the lungs to expand, pushing the heart away from the treatment area. This breath-hold action can reduce radiation received by the heart during radiotherapy.

Notes

17.3 Radical bladder

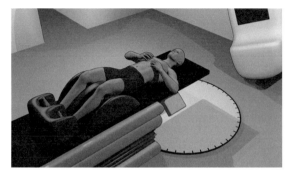

Beam arrangement

IMRT or VMAT moving 360° around the patient. Non-IMRT patients may have a four-field box arrangement.

Patient position

Supine, head to gantry, hands on chest.

Treatment preparation

Organ motion can be controlled by bladder and rectum preparation prior to each treatment.

Empty rectum (e.g. the patient may be asked to use a micro enema prior to each treatment) and to have a comfortable full bladder. This may be department-dependent. Please check the department's protocol.

Immobilisation devices

Stocks or Vac bag to secure the patient's feet, along with a knee support.

Typical prescriptions

64 Gy in 32# with 2 Gy/# over 6.5 weeks.

55 Gy in 20# with 2 Gy/# over 4 weeks.

> Radiographers need to check if the patient has undertaken their bladder or rectal preparations.

Some places will use Plan of the Day treatments, where a small, medium or large plan will be selected based on the day's IGRT imaging.

✎ Notes

_____

_____

_____

_____

_____

_____

_____

17.4 Radical lung

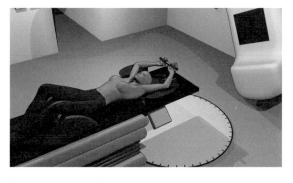

Beam arrangement

This arrangement varies greatly depending on the tumour location. IMRT or VMAT moving 360° around the patient.

Patient position

Supine, both arms raised above head holding onto the bar, elbows resting on the wings of the board. Knees slightly bent.

Immobilisation devices

A wing board is used with a T-bar attached; this is adjustable for each patient. A Vac bag may be used for additional support around the chest with a knee support. Patients may need to hold their breath with equipment (ABC) or breathe along with a metronome. Some places will have devices on the patient's abdomen to track their breathing in time.

Typical prescriptions

Lung SABR 18 Gy/ in 3# on alternate days

NSCLC – 55 Gy in 20# over 4 weeks.

66 Gy in 33# over 6.5 weeks.

SCLC – 40 Gy in 15# over 3 weeks.

Notes

17.5 Radical rectum

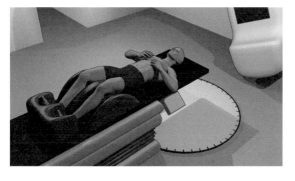

Beam arrangement

IMRT or VMAT moving 360° around the patient.

Patient position

Supine, head to gantry, hands on chest

Treatment preparation

Organ motion can be controlled by bladder and rectum preparation prior to each treatment.

Empty rectum (e.g. the patient may be asked to use a micro enema prior to each treatment) and to have a comfortable full bladder. This may be department-dependent. Please check the department's protocol.

Immobilisation devices

Knee support or Vac bag to secure feet, along with a knee support.

Typical prescription

45–50 Gy in 25# with 2 Gy/# over 5 weeks.

Reference: The Royal College of Radiologists (2019) *Radiotherapy Dose Fractionation*, 3rd edition. Available at: www.rcr.ac.uk/media/fezluddf/rcr-publications_radiotherapy-dose-fractionation-third-edition_march-2019.pdf.

✏️ Notes

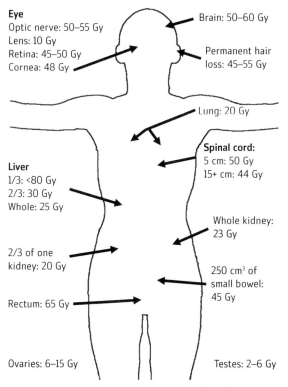

Eye
Optic nerve: 50–55 Gy
Lens: 10 Gy
Retina: 45–50 Gy
Cornea: 48 Gy

Brain: 50–60 Gy

Permanent hair loss: 45–55 Gy

Lung: 20 Gy

Spinal cord:
5 cm: 50 Gy
15+ cm: 44 Gy

Liver
1/3: <80 Gy
2/3: 30 Gy
Whole: 25 Gy

Whole kidney: 23 Gy

2/3 of one kidney: 20 Gy

250 cm³ of small bowel: 45 Gy

Rectum: 65 Gy

Ovaries: 6–15 Gy

Testes: 2–6 Gy

Reference: The Royal College of Radiologists (2019) *Radiotherapy Dose Fractionation*, 3rd edition. Available at: www.rcr.ac.uk/media/fezluddf/rcr-publications_radiotherapy-dose-fractionation-third-edition_march-2019.pdf.

19 | What is SABR?

- SABR can be used to treat primary lung tumours and metastatic tumours in the lungs, liver, bone (including spine), lymph nodes and adrenal glands that are smaller in size.
- Hypo-fractionation is used when delivering very high doses over 3, 5 or 8 fractions, resulting in increased chances of tumour control compared to conventional radiotherapy.
- It is used in conjunction with advanced motion managemen techniques such as 4DCT imaging and ABC, which helps to spare healthy tissue – minimising side-effects.
- It is suitable for patients who have been turned down for surgery due to tumour location or co-morbidities such as COPD, emphysema, heart problems or lung fibrosis.
- SABR is constantly evolving and in more recent years has been used in radical treatment; for example, prostate cancer.

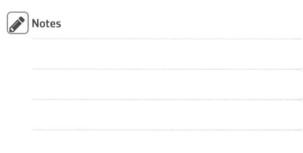 Notes

_____

_____

_____

_____

_____

Reference: Stereotactic radiotherapy | Cancer treatment | Cancer Research UK.

What is brachytherapy?

- 'Brachy' means 'short' in Greek so it is 'short therapy'.
- The radioactive substances are placed **directly into** or **very close** to the tumour.
- Radioactive materials or 'sources' include seeds, tubes and needles.
- The implant **can be left** for a period of time or permanently.
- A **higher dose** can be given to a **smaller area** compared with radiotherapy.
- Dose is given off **continuously**.
- The most common treatment you will come across using brachytherapy is for **prostate** cancer for men and **gynaecological** cancers in women.

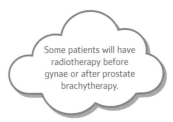

Some patients will have radiotherapy before gynae or after prostate brachytherapy.

Reference: Cancer Research UK (2020) *Cancer Treatments*. Available at: www.cancerresearchuk.org/about-cancer/treatment/radiotherapy.

- Electrons are used for **superficial** treatments.
- This can include skin cancers or a 'boost' to scar tissues.
- Very **minimal** side-effects, usually only erythema.
- This treatment does not usually have pre-planned gantry/collimator angles; skin apposition is used to set up the patient.
- Electrons **diverge** more than photons, which is why the applicator is so close to the patient's skin.
- The 'effective treatment depth' in cm is approximately 1/3 of the beam energy in MeV, e.g. 9 MeV treats to the effective depth of 3 cm.
- Different tissue densities, e.g. air and cartilage, can cause non-homogeneous (uneven) dose distributions.

When setting up the patient, an even skin apposition needs to be achieved (see *Chapter 22*). A lead cut-out can be placed into the applicator rather than placed on the patient for electron treatments. The applicator may come in contact with the patient's skin or have a gap, depending on department protocol.

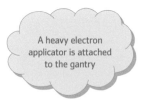

A heavy electron applicator is attached to the gantry

Reference: Barrett, A. *et al.* (2009) *Practical Radiotherapy Planning.* 4th ed. Taylor & Francis, p. 21.

What is orthovoltage and superficial X-ray therapy?

- Used for areas on/close to the **skin surface**, such as skin cancers.
- Orthovoltage uses a **higher energy** kilovoltage, whereas SXR (superficial X-ray) uses a **lower energy** kilovoltage treatment.
- The X-ray energy varies: up to 200 kV (kilovolts) for SXR and up to 500 kV for orthovoltage.
- It is not essential for the patient to lie on a hard carbon fibre bed. Instead they can sit or lie on a hospital bed, which makes this treatment more **comfortable**.
- The field shape and size is created by an **applicator** and a **lead cut-out**. A doctor will choose which shape and size to use during the planning stage.
- Lead shapes are also used for **extra shielding and immobilisation** of sensitive tissues, such as eyes. Lead stops the X-rays from penetrating the healthy skin.
- Immobilisation devices such as Vac bags (see *Chapter 3*) may be required for most patients, as the time to deliver treatment can be long. Typically this treatment is used on elderly patients who may find it harder to maintain their position throughout the treatment.
- This treatment is a '**free set-up**' so there are no set collimator or gantry angles. The radiographer will set the applicator so the distance between the applicator and the skin surface is as even as possible. This is known as '**skin apposition**'.
- Due to the size and shape of some cancers an even skin apposition can be difficult to achieve; there may be '**stand off**' or '**stand in**'.

- This set-up is similar for electron treatments. The main difference in set-up with electrons is that lasers and the FSD are used to achieve the correct distance between the applicator and skin.

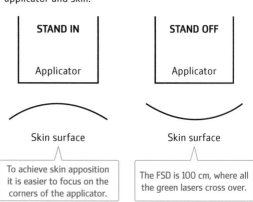

STAND IN

Applicator

Skin surface

To achieve skin apposition it is easier to focus on the corners of the applicator.

STAND OFF

Applicator

Skin surface

The FSD is 100 cm, where all the green lasers cross over.

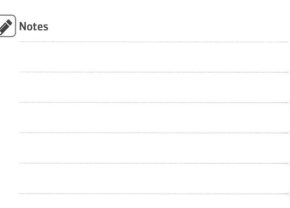

Notes

_____

_____

_____

_____

_____

_____

What is IGRT?

- IGRT stands for image-guided radiotherapy.
- IGRT is where the imaging is used to **increase the accuracy of treatment by reducing positional errors that can occur**.
- An image is taken on the treatment set and is **compared** with the image created when the patient was initially planned.
- Most departments will have different imaging protocols for each treatment site. Typically imaging is either daily or weekly. See your department's imaging protocol and ask questions.
- Imaging can be '**online**' or '**offline**'. Online is when the images are being checked just before the patient has their treatment, whilst offline is when a radiographer checks the images after the patient has had their treatment.
- Online imaging allows the radiographer to make small adjustments to the treatment couch before delivering the treatment. This will be only a matter of a few millimetres but will make it more accurate, and is known by radiographers as 'applying a move'. Most treatment machines can automatically move the patient to the correct position based on the imaging.
- Typically, a department's daily online imaging protocol will state to apply a shift over 1 mm.
- Typically, with weekly imaging, departments will have a margin where the image is:
  - **in tolerance**: the image matches the reference image enough to ensure accurate treatment.
  - **out of tolerance**: the image is not a close match to the reference image, and more imaging may be required. The moves made when setting up the patient may be altered slightly and checked with more imaging.

37

- **gross error**: it is not safe to treat because the patient's position is out of the safe margin to treat.

There are many different types of IGRT: 2DMV/kV, kV CBCT, MRI, US and 4DCBCT.

- **2DMV**: single image acquired before treatment. Treatment field defines image size. Only suitable if sufficient anatomy is visible. A double MV exposure can be used when insufficient anatomy is present in the treatment field to accurately assess set-up errors.
- **2DkV**: single image acquired before treatment. An image can be added to the treatment field, or alternatively a new angle can be created if found to be more useful. You can acquire two kV images (known as kV/kV paired) with 90° separation. The pair of 2D images are typically registered with the 3D reference data set. This means rotations can be analysed in 3D, therefore errors in all three directions can be corrected for.
- **Contrast** between bone and soft tissue is well defined with images acquired using kV imaging compared to images when using higher MV energies.
- **kV CBCT**: 3D volumetric data is obtained from the reconstruction of its 2D projections. These will be registered with the planning CT data set. CBCT allows the evaluation of bony structures as well as soft tissue, giving a more accurate verification which can be corrected prior to the treatment delivery.
- **MRI**: integrated with a treatment system aims to provide very high-quality soft tissue imaging for guidance before and during treatment delivery. MRI does not use ionising radiation.
- **US**: uses high-frequency sound to acquire images of internal structures. US images are acquired at pre-treatment and registered with the planning CT image and the radiotherapy-generated structure sets. US does not use ionising radiation.

- **4DCBCT**: 4DCBCT acquisition commonly sorts the projection images into the correct breathing state to provide a movie-loop style visualisation of respiratory motion. The scan requires more images therefore a longer scan time and a higher dose compared to conventional CBCT.

Top tip: prefixes and abbreviations

Prefix/suffix	Abbreviation	Multiple size
mega-	M	1,000,000
kilo-	k	1,000
milli-	m	0.001
-volts	V	–

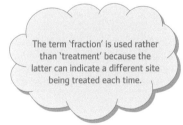

The term 'fraction' is used rather than 'treatment' because the latter can indicate a different site being treated each time.

Reference: The Royal College of Radiologists (2021) *On Target 2: updated guidance for image-guided radiotherapy*. Available at: www.rcr.ac.uk/our-services/all-our-publications/clinical-oncology-publications/on-target-2-updated-guidance-for-image-guided-radiotherapy.

24 | What is IMRT?

- IMRT stands for intensity-modulated radiotherapy.
- This is a technique used on most treatment sites.
- IMRT techniques alter the **intensity of the beam**, providing a **better dose distribution and tumour coverage** than conventional radiotherapy.
- The shape of the beam can be changed through the MLC (multi-leaf collimator). The MLC can move **continuously** while the treatment beam is being delivered, in either multiple beams or one continuous beam where the gantry rotates all around the patient.
- **VMAT** (volumetric arc therapy) is a term used when the gantry and MLCs are continuously moving around the patient. VMAT is an advanced radiotherapy technique that delivers the radiation dose continuously as the treatment machine rotates. This technique accurately shapes the radiation dose to the tumour while minimising the dose to organs around the tumour. This makes the treatment much more targeted and accurate than single beam-based radiotherapy.
- A reduced dose to normal tissues will result in fewer side-effects both in the short and long term. This improves the overall quality of life for the patient.
- Some IMRT treatments are quicker than conventional radiotherapy, especially if one continuous beam is used rather than multiple beams. The patient is thus on the treatment couch for less time, which gives a better patient experience than conventional radiotherapy.

Radiotherapy treatment pathway

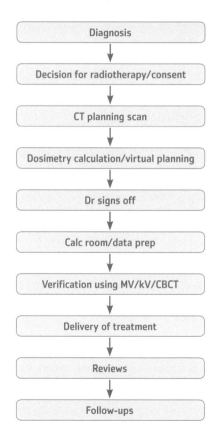

Diagnosis

↓

Decision for radiotherapy/consent

↓

CT planning scan

↓

Dosimetry calculation/virtual planning

↓

Dr signs off

↓

Calc room/data prep

↓

Verification using MV/kV/CBCT

↓

Delivery of treatment

↓

Reviews

↓

Follow-ups

Some patients may be put on hormone therapy. This treatment can be used to shrink or control tumours or reduce the risk of cancer returning. This is mostly used for breast and prostate cancers.

The main aims of hormone therapy are to lower oestrogen/testosterone levels or to block the receptors on the cancerous cell in order to starve it of the oestrogen/testosterone which encourages tumour growth.

Not all patients are able to have this treatment because it depends on the receptors present on the cells' surface.

The following is a list of some hormone therapy drugs used:

Brand name	Generic name	Application
Arimidex	Anastrozole	To treat breast cancer An aromatase inhibitor For post-menopausal women One tablet a day
Aromasin	Exemestane	To treat breast cancer For post-menopausal women An aromatase inhibitor One tablet a day
Casodex	Bicalutamide	To treat prostate cancer Injection or oral every 28 days
Zoladex	Goserelin	To treat breast and prostate cancer Injection, for 2 years For pre-menopausal women
Tamoxifen	Novadex	To treat breast cancer 20 mg Anti-oestrogen drug Adjuvant therapy taken for 5 years

What is immunotherapy?

- Immunotherapy uses the body's own immune system to recognise and attack cancer cells. It can be given in conjunction with chemotherapies and radiotherapy. There are different groups of immunotherapy called monoclonal antibodies or checkpoint inhibitors.
- Immunotherapy side-effects include inflammation anywhere in the body, most commonly of the bowel, skin, endocrine system and liver.
- Checkpoint inhibitor medications such as pembrolizumab, nivolumab and ipilimumab are main medications used for melanoma patients. These are given intravenously in the chemotherapy.
- Targeted therapies are used to block the growth of cancers. In melanoma we use encorafenib and binimetinib or dabrafenib and trametinib. They are all tablets that patients can take at home.

Notes

- Chemotherapy is a **systemic** treatment using a **cytotoxic** drug which involves the whole body.
- Chemotherapy may be one or a variety of drugs combined in a regime and 'cycles'.
- It can be administered either **intravenously, orally or topically**.
- Cancerous cells are continuously dividing by **mitosis**. Chemotherapy drugs **damage the cell's genes** when the cell is dividing, causing the cell to die.
- It can be used:
  - **to treat** any potential metastatic spread
  - **to shrink** the tumour for surgery or radiotherapy
  - as a sole **curative** treatment.
- Some treatments are time-sensitive, meaning radiotherapy has to be given within a certain time post-chemotherapy. Always check the department's protocol for these timings.
- Not all cancers are **sensitive** to chemotherapy.
- Patients with chemotherapy will experience **additional** side-effects. You should know what these are, so you can **differentiate** between chemotherapy and radiotherapy side-effects.

> Side-effects are caused by damage to normal cells; this is true for all treatments.

Reference: Cancer Research UK (2020) *Cancer Treatments*. Available at: www.cancerresearchuk.org/about-cancer/treatment/chemotherapy.

Chemotherapy side-effects

As with radiotherapy, individual patients will experience varying severity of side-effects. Each drug will have its own list of specific side-effects, and the patient will be made aware of these before they are asked for consent for treatment. The following are general side-effects of chemotherapy.

Side-effect	Details
Anaemia	Low red blood count, causing tiredness and fatigue
Hair loss	Hair follicles have a high cell turnover and are rapidly growing, so are targeted by the drug. Hair loss is reversible
Neutropenia	Low neutrophil cell count, weakened immune system, increased risk of infection
Nausea and vomiting	Steroids are usually given to help with nausea and to support appetite
Diarrhoea	This can be made worse by radiotherapy if treating the pelvic region
Dermatological toxicity	Some drugs can enhance reactions from radiotherapy such as cisplatin
Altered sense of taste	Some patients notice a metallic taste in their mouth or total loss of the sense of taste
Mucositis	Oral mucositis results from use of some chemotherapy drugs, because of the high cell turnover the drugs target

Most chemotherapy side-effects will fade away once treatment has stopped.

45

Skin reactions

Side-effects	Advice and medication
Erythema (mild reaction)	• Ensure the patient is not using any soaps/perfumes/deodorants which may contain metallic components. • Patients are advised to only use 'Simple' soap. • Moisturise twice a day with aqueous cream. Putting the cream in the fridge may help reduce the hot feeling. • Check the skin has not broken. • Loose-fitting clothing can reduce friction.
Dry desquamation (moderate reaction)	• Ensure that the patient is following the advice indicated above. • Fucibet (antibiotic cream) can be provided, to prevent infection. • If the patient has pruritus, 1% hydrocortisone can be prescribed. This should be given up to four times a day.
Moist desquamation (severe reaction)	• The patient must stop using the aqueous cream, and a dressing may be needed. • Hydrogel, which acts like another layer of skin, may be required. • Check with a swab to ensure the area is not infected.

See *Chapter 39* for a glossary on medical terminology.

 Note

> Skin reactions are worse in areas where skin folds cause friction, for example, under the breast.

Brain and central nervous system

Side-effects	Advice and medication
• Raised intracranial pressure causing headaches, nausea, blurred vision and an unsteady gait • Tiredness • Dysphasia • Hair loss	• Ensure the patient is drinking plenty of fluids • Dexamethasone: a steroid which can be prescribed to reduce the intracranial pressure • Metoclopramide: an antiemetic for nausea

Neck and thorax

Side-effects	Advice and medication
• Pain • Dysphagia • Mucositis • Xerostomia • Weight loss • Hair loss • Fungal infection • Haemoptysis • Breathlessness	• Refer patient to the dietitian and speech and language therapist if problems persist. Nutritional drinks can be provided in order to reduce the weight loss. • Analgesics such as paracetamol and morphine are provided to help the patient swallow soft food more easily. • General advice such as avoiding alcohol and spicy foods and stopping smoking will help reduce side-effects. • Nystatin: prevents any fungal infection. • Difflam: treats mucositis. • Artificial saliva: for xerostomia. • Antacid: helps with dysphagia.

Breast

Side-effects	Advice and medication
• Pain • Tiredness • Severe skin reaction	• Skin reaction can be worse due to friction. It should be suggested that the patient wears a non-wired bra with loose-fitting clothing, whilst still following the skin care advice. • Analgesics such as paracetamol can be provided to reduce the pain/heaviness.

Pelvic region

Side-effects	Advice and medication
• Difficulty in micturition • Cystitis • Haematuria • Proctitis • Diarrhoea • Tiredness	• A mid-stream urine (MSU) sample should be taken to ensure the cystitis is radiation-induced and not due to infection. • Information on appropriate diet should be given, including advice on eating less fibre. • Loperamide: relieves diarrhoea if dietary changes fail.

References:

Breast: Macmillan Cancer Support (2018) *Radiotherapy for Breast Cancer*. Available at: www.macmillan.org.uk/cancer-information-and-support/treatments-and-drugs/radiotherapy-for-breast-cancer.

Brain/CNS: Macmillan Cancer Support (2019) *Radiotherapy for a Brain Tumour*. Available at: www.macmillan.org.uk/cancer-information-and-support/treatments-and-drugs/radiotherapy-for-a-brain-tumour.

Pelvis:

• Macmillan Cancer Support (2020) *Radiotherapy for Anal Cancer*. Available at: www.macmillan.org.uk/cancer-information-and-support/treatments-and-drugs/radiotherapy-for-anal-cancer.

• Macmillan Cancer Support (2021a) *Radiotherapy for Cervical Cancer*. Available at: www.macmillan.org.uk/cancer-information-and-support/treatments-and-drugs/radiotherapy-for-cervical-cancer.

• Macmillan Cancer Support (2021b). *Radiotherapy for Prostate Cancer*. Available at: www.macmillan.org.uk/cancer-information-and-support/treatments-and-drugs/radiotherapy-for-prostate-cancer.

Head & neck: Macmillan Cancer Support (2022) *Side Effects of Radiotherapy for Head and Neck Cancer*. Available at: www.macmillan.org.uk/cancer-information-and-support/head-and-neck-cancer/side-effects-of-radiotherapy-for-head-and-neck-cancer.

Notes

Some patients will undergo a weekly blood test to ensure that they are not anaemic, as this will affect the effectiveness of radiotherapy. Anaemia is when the patient's haemoglobin levels are low; haemoglobin in red blood cells carries the oxygen, and when there is less haemoglobin and therefore less oxygen in the body, cells can be hypoxic. Hypoxic cells are radio-resistant, therefore radiotherapy is not as effective. If the haemoglobin level becomes too low, a blood transfusion may be required.

A blood test can also monitor the white blood count, as this can indicate if the patient is immunosuppressed or has a possible infection.

Haematology	Male	Female
White blood cell (WBC)	$4–11 \times 10^9/L$	$4–11 \times 10^9/L$
Red blood cell (RBC)	$4.5–6.5 \times 10^{12}/L$	$3.8–5 \times 10^{12}/L$
Haemoglobin (Hb)	13–18 g/mL	12–16 g/mL
Neutrophil	$2.0–7.5 \times 10^9/L$	$2.0–7.5 \times 10^9/L$
Platelets (thrombocytes)	$150–440 \times 10^9/L$	$150–440 \times 10^9/L$

References: Longmore, M. *et al.* (2014) *Oxford Handbook of Clinical Medicine*. Oxford University Press.

Waugh, A. & Grant, A. (2005) *Ross and Wilson: Anatomy and Physiology in Health and Illness*. Churchill Livingstone. 9th ed

Cancer Research UK (2022) *Blood Tests*. Available at: www. cancerresearchuk.org/about-cancer/tests-and-scans/blood-tests

Radiotherapy manufacturers

There are two main manufacturers of equipment within radiotherapy: Varian and Elekta. They both make linear accelerators (Linac) that can deliver high energy X-rays or electrons to conform to a tumour's shape and destroy cancer cells while sparing surrounding normal tissue. Although both deliver the same outcome, there are a few differences between them.

- **Hand pendants**: Varian has two hand pendants at the end of the bed, whereas Elekta has two hand pendants on the wall, either side of the Linac. Additionally, they both have bed controls. The controls on the pendants are different; therefore, take your time to familiarise yourself with them while on placement. If you have any free time between patients don't be afraid to ask if you can go into the room to do so.
- **Computer software**: Varian operates with ARIA and Elekta operates with Mosaiq software. These systems manage the treatment process; for example patient appointments, treatment records and electronic documentation.

Notes

Skull

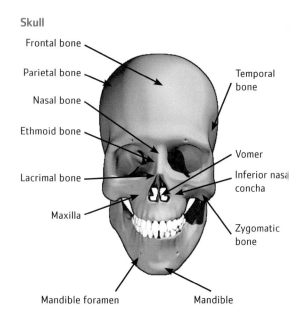

- Frontal bone
- Parietal bone
- Nasal bone
- Ethmoid bone
- Lacrimal bone
- Maxilla
- Temporal bone
- Vomer
- Inferior nasal concha
- Zygomatic bone
- Mandible foramen
- Mandible

 Notes

Pelvis

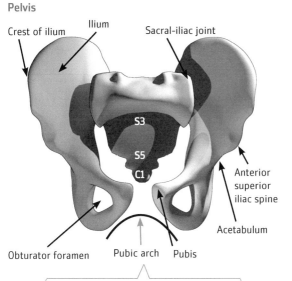

Crest of ilium

Ilium

Sacral-iliac joint

S3

S5

C1

Anterior superior iliac spine

Acetabulum

Obturator foramen

Pubic arch

Pubis

The pubic arch is more V shaped in men than women; this image is based on a male pelvis.

Notes

C1:   Base of skull, hard palate

C3:   Angle of mandible, hyoid bone, epiglottis

C4:   Thyroid cartilage, thyroid upper level

C6:   Cricoid cartilage, pharynx, isthmus of thyroid gland

T2:   Sternal notch

T3:

T4:   Sternal angle carina (bifurcation of trachea)

T5:

T9:   Xiphisternal joint

T10:   Oesophagus enters diaphragm

T11:   Oesophagus enters stomach

T12:   Abdominal aorta

L1:   Spinal cord, foramen magnum, renal arteries

L2:   Gall bladder

L3:   Umbilicus, lower costal margin

L4:   Umbilicus, iliac crest, bifurcation of abdominal aorta

Larynx:	C3–C6
Trachea:	C6–T4
Oesophagus:	C6–T11 (22 cm long)
Aortic arch:	2.5 cm below suprasternal notch–T4
Stomach:	T4–T10
Spleen:	9th rib–11th rib
Right kidney:	T11–L3
Pancreas:	L1–2
Left kidney:	T11–L3
Pulmonary artery:	Arises at 2nd costal cartilage, Bifurcates at 3rd left costal cartilage
Liver:	5th costal space – 10th costal space
Rectum:	Line joining posterior superior iliac crest – S3
Pituitary gland:	2.5 cm Ant + 2.5 cm Sup to tragus
Parotid:	Extends from tragus – 2 cm below angle of mandible
Pineal gland:	3 cm Sup + 1.5 cm Post of tragus

Notes

Note

> Good manual handling is essential in order to prevent injury to yourself and others.

✓	✗
Bending your knees when lifting/putting down objects	Having a stooped back when picking up heavy objects
Keeping the heavy load close to your body	Rushing and not asking for additional help with awkward/heavy loads
Having a stable base at all times	Bending and twisting at the same time
Using a 'rocking' motion when assisting a patient to stand up, ensuring that they move to the edge of their seat first	Allowing the patient to hold onto you in order to pull themselves up
Not undertaking strain on your back unnecessarily	Not clearing a pathway when moving a load or patient
Using aids such as a pat-slide and a slide sheet	Using equipment which has an out-of-date service check
Keeping your head up when carrying loads	Not applying the brakes to movable equipment, e.g. a wheelchair

 Notes

Infection control

Hand washing is important in order to prevent the spread of infection to staff and patients.

Some patients may be immunosuppressed due to chemotherapy treatments, therefore great care and attention should be given to hand hygiene.

When should I wash my hands?

- Before touching the patient
- When leaving the treatment room in between beams
- After each time you touch the patient
- After any contact with bodily fluid (you should be wearing gloves for this too)
- After the patient has had their treatment.

What should I use to wash my hands?

For the times you are in a hurry, for example when leaving the room to switch on, **alcohol gel** should be provided in dispensers on the walls to quickly use on the way out. You shouldn't use this every time; in between patients **soap and warm water** is more appropriate. Do not use alcohol gel when your hands are visibly dirty.

Tip

> On the walls by a sink there should be a poster instructing you on how to wash your hands most effectively.

57

In an emergency dial '2222' in order to call the crash team. Tell the operator if the patient is a child or an adult and if possible have the patient's notes at hand to help the crash team.

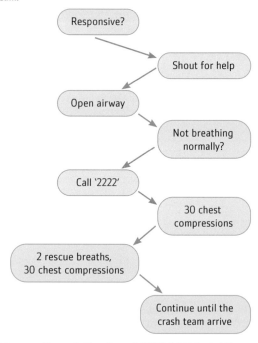

Reference: Resuscitation Council (2021) *Adult Basic Life Support*. Available at: www.resus.org.uk/library/2021-resuscitation-guidelines/adult-basic-life-support-guidelines.

The recovery position

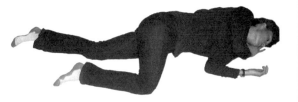

Points to remember

- Ensure the airway is open by keeping their head tilted back – adjusting their hand may help you with this.
- Check their breathing regularly.
- If the patient is still in the recovery position after 30 minutes, put them into the recovery position on their other side.
- NEVER put anything in their mouth.
- NEVER move the patient unless instructed to do so.

Notes

Reference: St John Ambulance [online] *How to put an adult in the recovery position*. Available at: www.sja.org. uk/get-advice/first-aid-advice/unresponsive-casualty/ how-to-do-the-recovery-position.

Acute toxicity: side-effects which occur immediately or shortly after treatment. In general these side-effects reduce over time.

Adenocarcinoma: cancer of a gland or glandular tissue, which arises in the epithelium.

Adenoma: a benign tumour.

Adjuvant treatment: treatment given in addition to the primary treatment to increase long-term survival.

Analgesic: drugs used to relieve pain.

Antiemetic drug: used to treat nausea and vomiting.

Asymptomatic: without symptoms.

Benign: non-cancerous tumours that do not invade or destroy local tissues and do not spread to other sites in the body.

Biopsy: a diagnostic test in which a small amount of tissue or cells are removed from the body for microscopic examination.

Carcinoma: any cancerous tumour arising from cells in the covering surface layer or lining membrane of an organ.

Carcinoma *in situ*: the earliest stage of a cancer in which it has not yet spread from the surface layer of cells of an organ.

Catheter: a flexible tube inserted into the body to drain or introduce fluids.

Cystitis: inflammation of the bladder lining.

Dysphagia: difficulty swallowing.

Dysphasia: inability to select the words with which to speak and write.

Erythema: redness of the skin.

Fractionation: dividing the total dose of radiation into smaller doses conventionally given once a day.

Haematuria: blood in urine.

Haemoptysis: coughing up blood.

Hyperfractionation: increasing the number of fractions compared to conventional treatment. This decreases the dose per fraction.

Hypofractionation: decreasing the number of fractions compared to conventional treatment. This increases the dose per fraction.

Lumpectomy: surgical treatment for breast cancer in which only the cancer tissue is removed.

Malignant: cancerous tumour that spreads from its original location to form secondary tumour in other parts of the body.

Mastectomy: surgical removal of the entire breast.

Metastasis: a secondary tumour which has spread from a primary tumour in another part of the body.

Micturition: passing urine.

Mucus: thick slimy fluid secreted by mucous membranes.

Neoadjuvant: treatment given in addition to the primary treatment but administered prior to primary treatment.

Palliative treatment: treatment of any type that is intended to relieve the signs and symptoms of cancer and improve the patient's quality of life.

Proctitis: inflammation of the rectum.

Prostatectomy: an operation to remove part or all of the prostate gland.

Radical treatment: treatment of any type which is intended to cure the cancer.

Xerostomia: dryness of the mouth.

Notes

References: The British Medical Association (BMA) (2018) *Illustrated Medical Dictionary*. 4th ed. London: Dorling Kindersley, p. 501.

McArdle, O. and O'Mahony, D. (2008) *Oncology*. London: Churchill Livingstone, pp. 119–120.

My Notes

My Notes